STEM and COVID-19

by Grace Hansen

Dr. Anthony Richie as Content Consultant

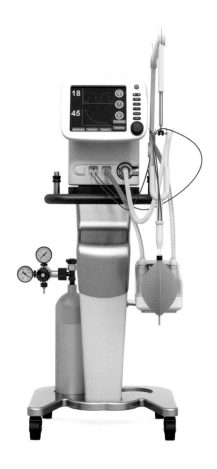

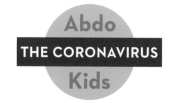

Abdo Kids Jumbo is an Imprint of Abdo Kids
abdobooks.com

abdobooks.com

Published by Abdo Kids, a division of ABDO, P.O. Box 398166, Minneapolis, Minnesota 55439.
Copyright © 2021 by Abdo Consulting Group, Inc. International copyrights reserved in all countries.
No part of this book may be reproduced in any form without written permission from the publisher.
Abdo Kids Jumbo™ is a trademark and logo of Abdo Kids.

Printed in the United States of America, North Mankato, Minnesota.

052020

092020

THIS BOOK CONTAINS
RECYCLED MATERIALS

Photo Credits: Alamy, AP Images, Getty Images, iStock, Science Source, Shutterstock

Production Contributors: Teddy Borth, Jennie Forsberg, Grace Hansen
Design Contributors: Dorothy Toth, Pakou Moua

Library of Congress Control Number: 2020936730

Publisher's Cataloging-in-Publication Data

Names: Hansen, Grace, author.

Title: STEM and COVID-19 / by Grace Hansen

Description: Minneapolis, Minnesota : Abdo Kids, 2021 | Series: The Coronavirus | Includes online
    resources and index.

Identifiers: ISBN 9781098205553 (lib. bdg.) | ISBN 9781098205690 (ebook) | ISBN 9781098205768
    (Read-to-Me ebook)

Subjects: LCSH: Immunotechnology--Juvenile literature. | Medical technology--Juvenile literature. |
    Biomedical research--Juvenile literature. | Epidemics--Juvenile literature. | Communicable diseases--
    Prevention--Juvenile literature. | Health--Juvenile literature.

Classification: DDC 610.28--dc23

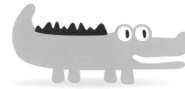

Table of Contents

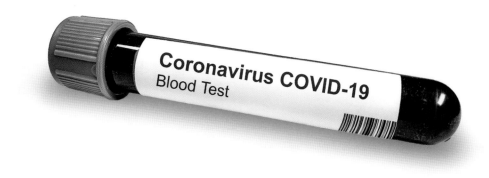

STEM & COVID-19

During the COVID-19 outbreak, scientists and **engineers** worked hard. Their work continues to save lives today.

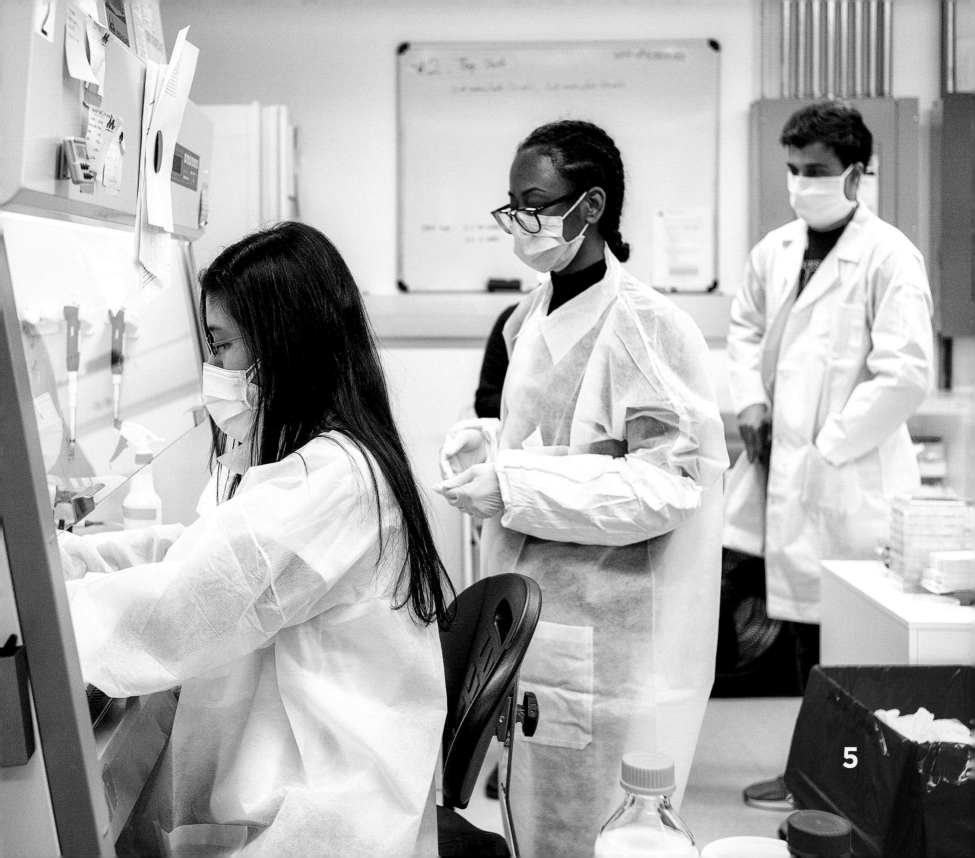

COVID-19 is an illness caused by a certain coronavirus. Most people with COVID-19 get a cough and fever. Others can have trouble breathing and even die.

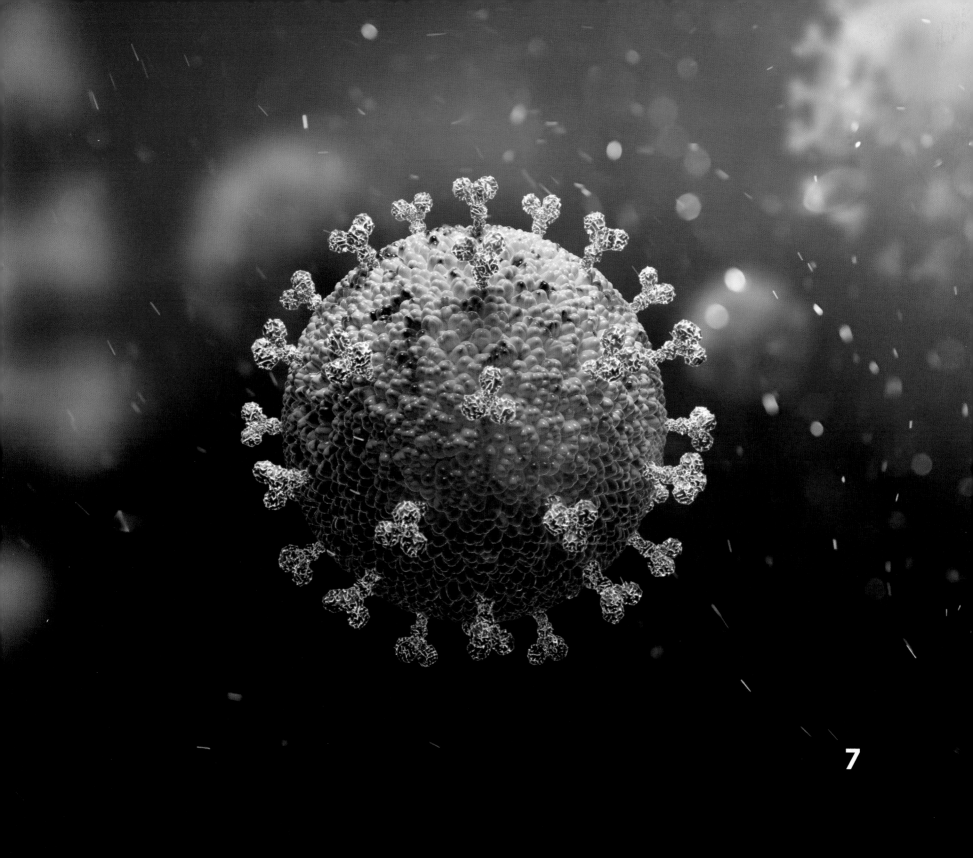

7

STEM that Saves Lives

COVID-19 can attack people's lungs. A ventilator is needed if a patient's lungs are failing. This amazing machine breathes for them.

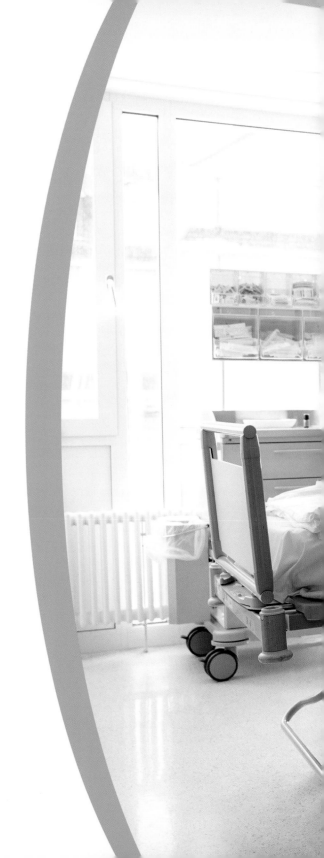

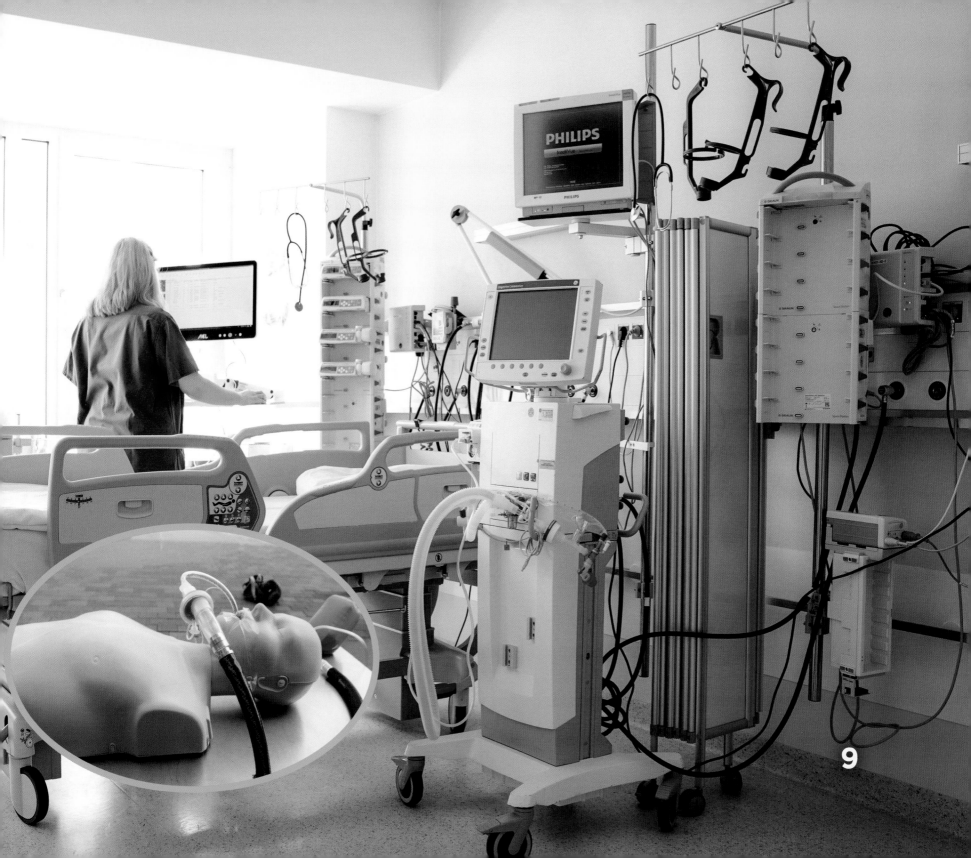

Fast lab testing for COVID-19 is necessary. The more people we test, the more information we have. The information is used to keep the **virus** from spreading. This saves lives!

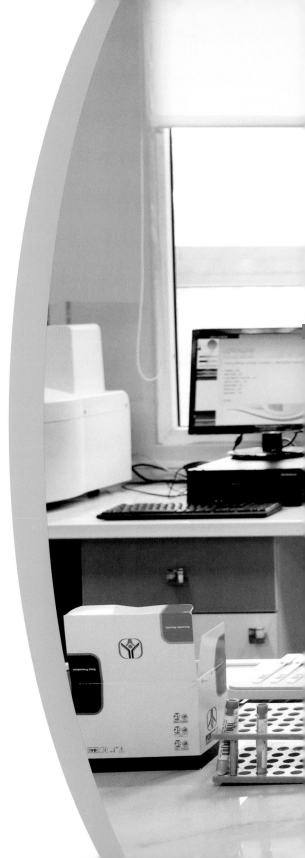

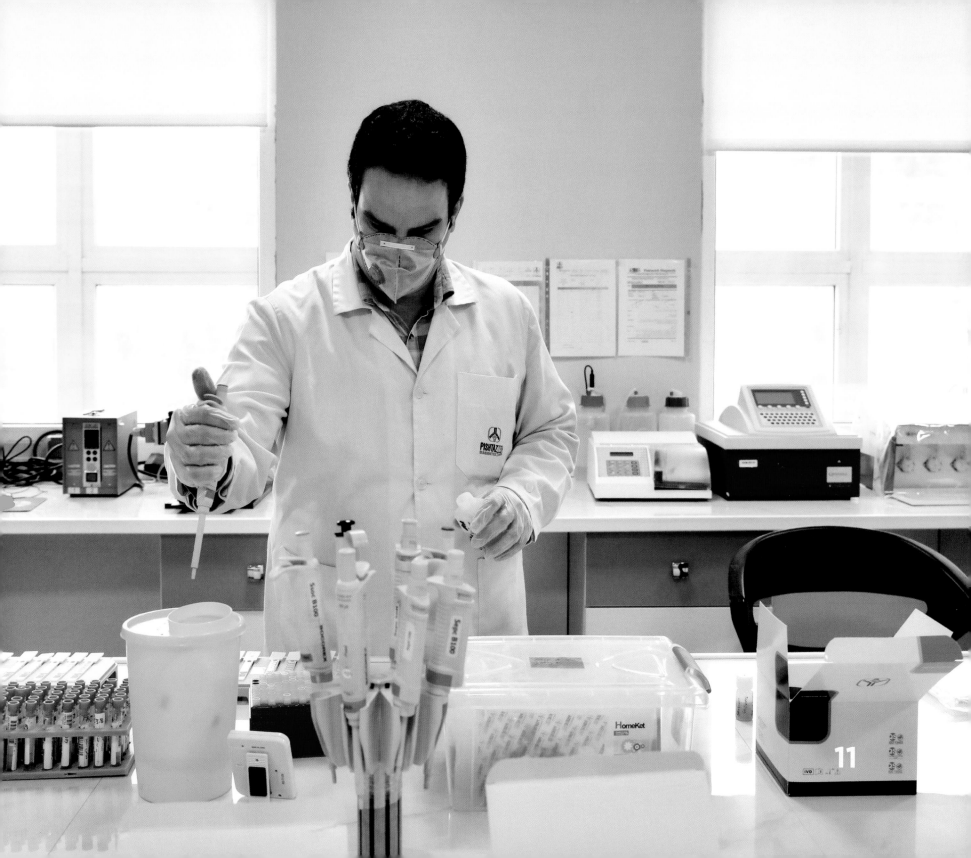

Finding a vaccine is also important to save lives. A vaccine contains the **virus** that causes an illness. The virus is either weakened or killed. It cannot make you sick.

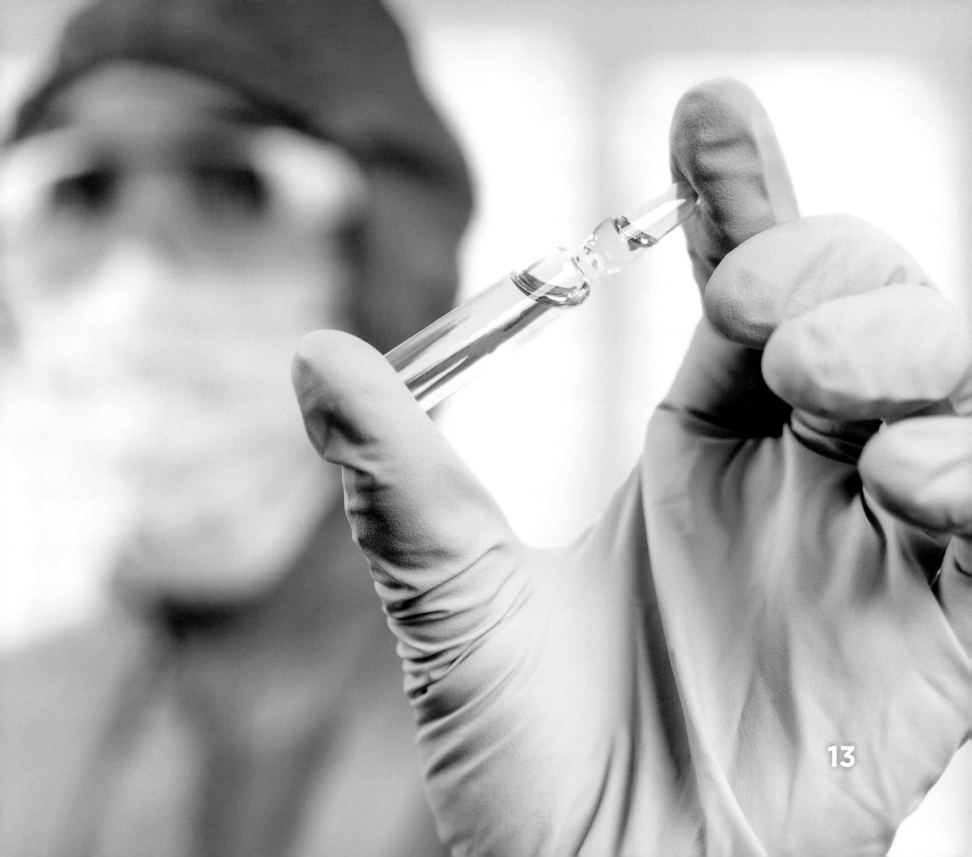

Vaccines introduce your **immune system** to a **virus**. Your immune system makes **antibodies** to fight it.

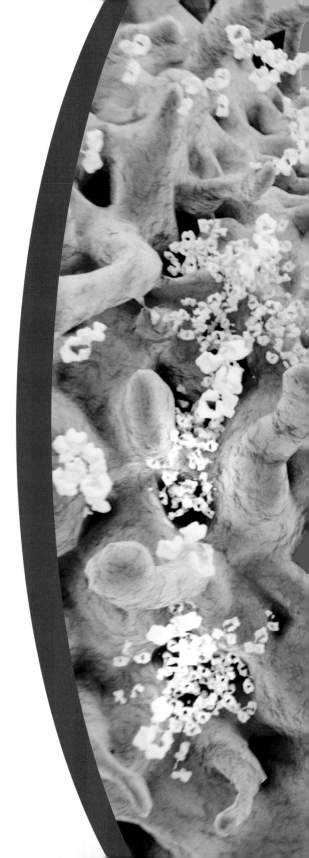

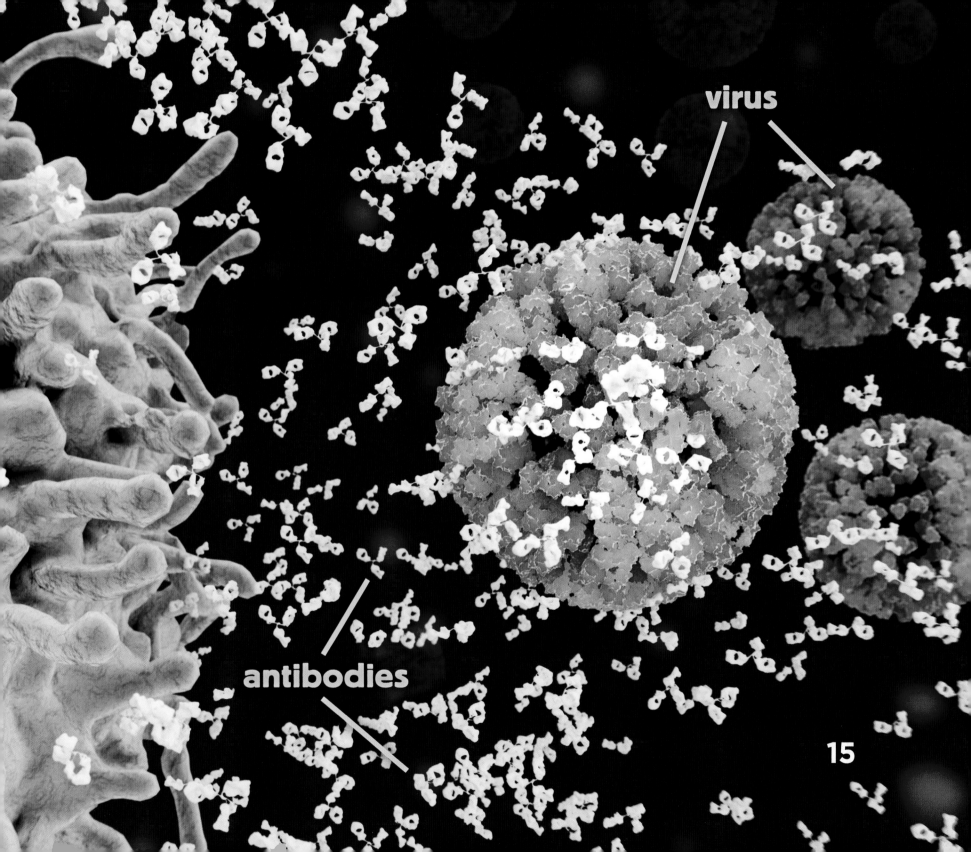

virus

antibodies

15

People who have recovered from COVID-19 can also help. Their **immune systems** have made **antibodies** that fight the **virus**. These antibodies can be given to people who are sick.

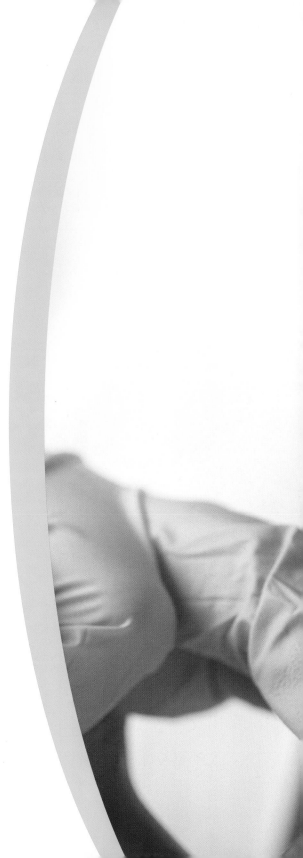

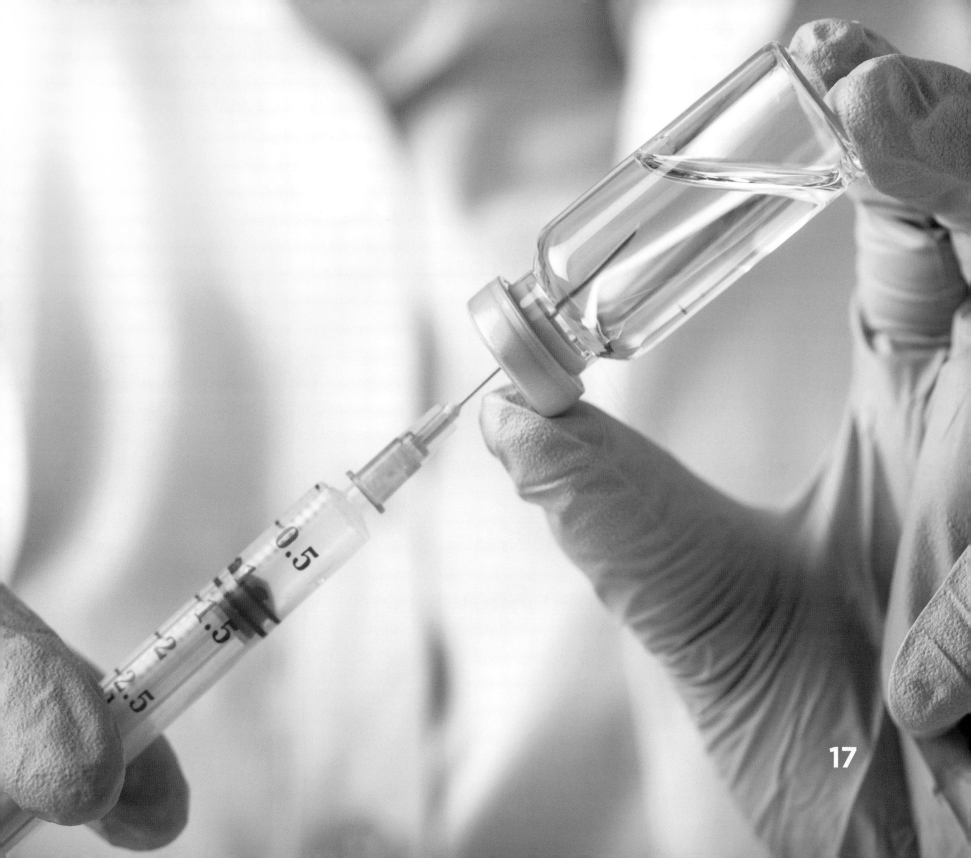

During a health crisis, drones are for more than just fun. They can bring medical supplies to hospitals. They deliver medicine to people who can't leave their homes.

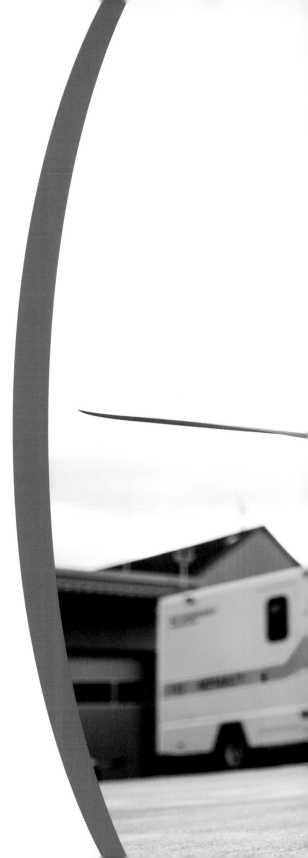

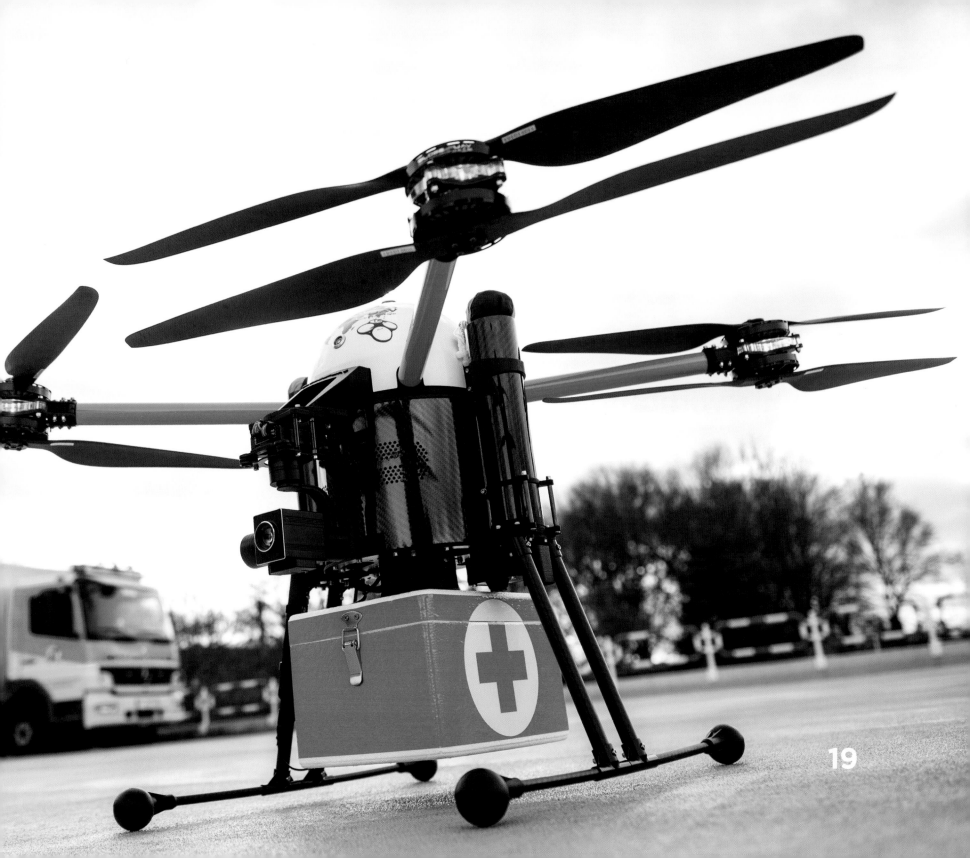

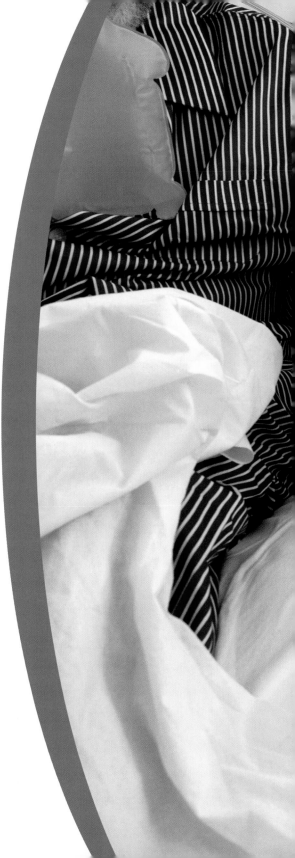

Health care robots help in COVID-19 patient care. Robots allow doctors to talk to the patients without being in the room. Robots can check people's **vitals**, like blood pressure and temperature. They can even clean hospitals.

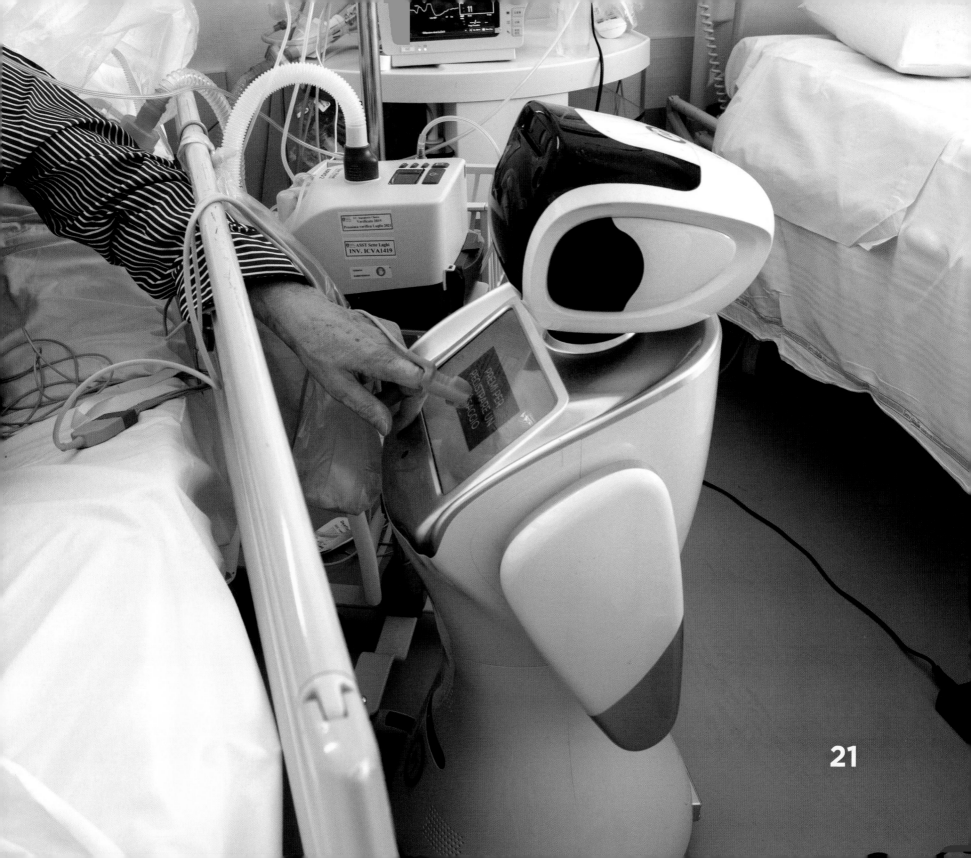

21

More Information About COVID-19

- COVID-19 is short for <u>Co</u>rona<u>v</u>irus <u>D</u>isease 20<u>19</u>.

- COVID-19 is an illness caused by a coronavirus strain called SARS-CoV-2.

- SARS-CoV-2 is short for Severe Acute Respiratory Syndrome Coronavirus 2.

- Common symptoms of COVID-19 include cough, fever, and shortness of breath.

Glossary

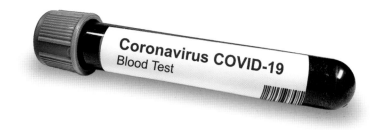

antibody – a protein in blood that reacts to viruses by neutralizing or destroying them. Antibodies provide immunity against viruses.

coronavirus – one in a group of viruses that cause disease. In humans, coronaviruses cause respiratory tract infections, like the common cold or a more deadly illness.

engineer – one who is trained in the use or design of machines or other technologies.

immune system – the bodily system which protects the body by detecting the presence of, and destroying, disease-causing viruses.

virus – a tiny organism that can reproduce only in living cells. Viruses can cause illnesses in humans, animals, and plants.

vitals – also known as vital signs, a group of the most important medical signs, like pulse, temperature, and blood pressure, that show the status of the body's life-sustaining functions.

23

Index

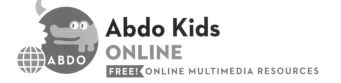

Visit **abdokids.com**
to access crafts, games,
videos, and more!

Use Abdo Kids code
TSK5553
or scan this QR code!

24